Achieving Your Ideal Skin

An Easy Guide to Daily Self-Care

E. Peter

Table of Contents

Introduction

A consistent skincare routine can improve specific skin concerns, such as acne, scars, and dark spots, while also promoting overall skin health, regardless of skin type.

Knowing your skin type is crucial when selecting skincare products. Although you may think your skin is either sensitive, oily, or dry, do you know what your actual skin type is? It's important to determine your skin type before heading to the cosmetics aisle to avoid using the wrong products, which could exacerbate dryness, acne, or other skin issues. Even some popular online skincare hacks may not be suitable for your skin type, so identifying your skin type is essential for achieving healthy and radiant skin.

Chapter 1

Building a daily skincare routine

A daily skincare routine consists of four fundamental procedures that you can perform once in the morning and once before going to bed.

1. **Cleansing:** Choose a cleanser that does not dry out your skin after washing. If you have dry skin and don't wear makeup, clean your face no more than twice a day. Washing for that squeaky-clean feeling is bad since it removes your skin's natural oils.

2. **Moisturizer:** Even oily skin needs moisturizing; however, choose a product that doesn't clog pores, is lightweight, gel-based, and non-comedogenic. More moisturizers with a cream basis could be beneficial for dry skin. Most manufacturers will indicate on the packaging whether their product is a gel or a cream.

A quick look at the best moisturizers for dry skin

- **Best gentle moisturizer for dry skin:** NIVEA Soft Moisturizing Creme
- Eucerin Advanced Repair Cream is the best moisturizer for skin that is rough, damaged, and scaly.
- Andalou Naturals Purple Carrot + C Luminous Night Cream is the best affordable face moisturizer.
- **Best moisturizer for sensitive skin:** Kiehl's Ultra Facial Cream
- **Best oil-free moisturizer:** CeraVe Moisturizing Cream
- **Best moisturizer for acne-prone skin:** Rael Miracle Clear Barrier Cream
- The best moisturizer for the entire body is Eufora Aloetherapy Moisture Mist.

Moisturizers of high quality can assist to soothe and restore dry, itchy, and irritated skin. A moisturizer is an integral component of any skin care regimen. It helps to keep your skin's moisture barrier intact and protects it from environmental damage.

A daily lightweight moisturizer filled with hydrating ingredients like niacinamide or hyaluronic acid can help alleviate dry or dull skin.

A quick look at the best moisturizers for oily skin

- **Best for acne:** Origins Clear Improvement Moisturizer
- **Best fragrance-free formula:** BeautyStat Universal Pro-Bio Moisture Boost Cream
- **Best anti-aging formula**: Peter Thomas Roth Water Drench Hyaluronic Cloud Cream Hydrating Moisturizer.
- **Best lightweight moisturizer:** SkinMedica Ultra Sheer Moisturizer
- **Best moisturizer with SPF**: Cetaphil Pro Oil Absorbing Moisturizer
- **Best overall:** Neutrogena Hydro Boost Gel-Cream

If you have oily skin, you might have noticed that your T-zone gets shiny and you experience acne breakouts.

Even though it may seem counterintuitive, including a moisturizer in your skincare routine is crucial, especially if you have excess oil.

Products that you use frequently to treat acne and outbreaks may be depleting your skin's natural oils. Your face may overcompensate by creating extra oil as a result, which might potentially cause dryness and irritation in the process.

A quick look at the best moisturizers for sensitive skin

- **Best gel moisturizer:** Aveeno Calm + Restore Oat Gel Moisturizer.
- **Best vegan formula:** Youth to the People Superfood Air-Whip Moisture Cream
- **Best for acne-prone skin:** Neutrogena Oil-Free Moisturizer with Sunscreen
- **Best for mature-looking skin:** Kate Somerville Age Arrest Anti-Wrinkle Cream
- One of the best drugstore finds is Simple Kind to Skin Replenishing Moisturiser.
- Best overall: CeraVe Moisturizing Cream

Your skin deserves to look and feel its best, and that's why it's important to keep it moisturized. If you have sensitive skin, don't let that stop you from finding the right products. With a little patience and effort, you can discover the perfect skincare routine that will make you feel confident and beautiful.

3. **Serums:** In the morning, it is preferable to use a serum containing growth factors, peptides, or vitamin C under sunscreen, while retinol or prescription retinoids work best at night.

A quick look at the best face serums for every skin type

Best for oily skin

- The Ordinary Niacinamide 10% + Zinc 1%
- SkinCeuticals Retexturing Activator
- Peach & Lily Glass Skin Refining Serum

Best for sensitive skin

- EltaMD Skin Recovery Face Serum
- Krave Beauty Great Barrier Relief

- Mad Hippie Vitamin A Serum
- **Best for dry, acne-prone skin**
- The INKEY List Hyaluronic Acid Hydrating Serum
- Farmacy Honeymoon Glow AHA Resurfacing Night Serum
- First Aid Beauty Ultra Repair® Hydrating Serum

Best for aging skin

- The INKEY List Retinol Anti-Aging Serum
- SkinCeuticals C E Ferulic Combination Antioxidant Treatment
- Biossance Squalane + Copper Peptide Rapid Plumping Serum

Best for combination skin

- Paula's Choice Omega+ Complex Serum
- Tata Harper Resurfacing AHA + BHA Serum
- Glow Recipe Avocado Ceramide Redness Relief Serum.

If you're in search of a skincare product that you can use after cleansing but before moisturizing, then a serum would be a great option. Generally, serums have a liquid consistency and leave little residue, making them ideal for layering.

They contain more potent concentrations of active ingredients, like hyaluronic acid, vitamin C, niacinamide, and more.

4. **Sunscreen:** It is recommended to apply sunscreen with at least 30 SPF 15 minutes before going outdoors since it takes time for sunscreen to be effective. People with darker skin tones require more sun protection because hyperpigmentation is more difficult to treat.

Make sure the items you choose suit your skin type and sensitivity level by carefully reading the labels.

7 Best Sunscreens for Face, Recommended by Dermatologists

Sun protection is essential for preventing wrinkles, sun spots, acne scarring, and skin cancer. Some experts claim that a skincare routine is pointless without sun protection. Therefore, it's crucial to apply the best sunscreen for your face. However, finding the right sunscreen can be challenging.

To help you find the best face sunscreens for every skin type, we polled dermatologists for their top picks including:

- **Best for Mature Skin:** sonage Roux Tinted Day Creme with SPF 30, $60
- **Best for Oily Skin:** Hero Cosmetics Force Shield Superlight Sunscreen, $18
- **Best for Sensitive Skin:** Blue Lizard Sensitive Face Mineral Sunscreen, $17
- **Best Drugstore Facia Sunscreen:** Neutrogena Ultra Sheer Dry-Touch Water Resistant and Non-Greasy Sunscreen, $13

- ❖ **Best for every day:** Doctor Babor Protect RX Mineral Sunscreen SPF 30, $53

- ❖ **Best Tinted Sunscreen:** Tower 28 SunnyDays SPF 30 Tinted Sunscreen Foundation, $32

- ❖ **Best Overall SPF for Face:** EltaMD UV Sport Broad Spectrum SPF 50, $30

Do this for all skin types

- Stay hydrated.
- Change pillowcases at least once a week.
- Wash or wrap up hair before bed.
- Wear sunscreen every day and apply 15 minutes before going out.

It's better to start with a simple routine to gauge your skin's reaction. Once you feel comfortable, you can add more products such as masks, exfoliants, and spot treatments to enhance your skin's health.

Remember to patch-test new products as well, particularly if you think you may have sensitive skin. You can use this to detect possible allergic reactions.

To patch-test a new product:

Apply a small amount of product on your skin in a discreet area, such as the inside of your wrist or your inner arm.

Wait 48 hours to see if there's a reaction.

Check the area 96 hours after application to see if you have a delayed reaction.

If you experience itching, redness, discomfort, or tiny pimples, it may be a sign of an allergic reaction. In this case, wash the affected area with water and a mild cleanser. You should return the product and select one that is more appropriate for your skin type.

Chapter 2

Treatment options for skin issues

There are methods for treating skin issues without endangering your skin. But always keep in mind the most important rule for skin care: Don't pick!

It's not recommended to pick at skin conditions such as blackheads, scabs, or acne as it may lead to hyperpigmentation, the darkening of skin areas, or open wounds. Open wounds can cause scars, increased acne, or infections. Keep in mind that the deeper the wound, the more likely it is to leave a scar on your skin.

These are a few treatments for problem areas that have scientific support.

1. Acne

Effective acne treatment depends on the severity of acne. For mild acne, nonprescription products from local drugstores can be used alongside overall skin care such as:

- tea tree oil

- benzoyl peroxide

- alpha hydroxy acids

- salicylic acid

What causes acne?

When dead skin cells, germs, and sebum are all stuck in a hair follicle, the result is clogged pores, which is the usual cause of acne.

Every pore present on the surface of the skin is an opening to a hair follicle, which comprises hair and an oil gland. When the oil gland functions correctly, it secretes sebum that travels up through the hair and comes out of the pore. The sebum then reaches the skin, where its primary function is to keep the skin lubricated.

If something goes wrong during this process, acne could appear.

Acne is directly caused by the blockage of skin pores due to excessive sebum, dead skin cells, or bacteria accumulation.

How can you determine which treatment is best for you?

Depending on the kind and severity of your acne, you can choose the appropriate treatment for it.

According to Julie C. Harper, MD, a board-certified dermatologist and clinical associate professor of dermatology at the University of Alabama-Birmingham, the only reliable way to determine the right acne treatment plan is to consult with a dermatology provider. "Bear in mind that acne comes in various forms and treatment regimens vary from one person to another," she emphasizes. Therefore, seeking professional advice is crucial to achieving clearer and healthier skin.

A dermatologist will closely examine your skin to see which of the different types of lesions appear:

- ➢ Moderate inflammatory acne includes papules and pustules.
- ➢ Mild noninflammatory acne (aka comedonal acne) includes whiteheads and blackheads.

Non-inflammatory acne is often treatable with OTC products containing active ingredients like salicylic acid and benzoyl peroxide or prescription-strength topical retinoids.

A dermatologist's prescription is needed for topical or oral medications for inflammatory acne.

While OTC products can help with papules and pustules, inflammatory acne requires a dermatologist to prevent scarring.

2. Sebaceous filaments

Sebaceous filaments are small, whitish-yellow tubes that resemble cylinders inside your pores. These are frequently mistaken for blackheads, which are merely an oxidized form of acne.

Sebaceous filaments are tiny collections of sebum and dead skin cells that can be found in your pores. They can make your pores appear larger than they are, which can be frustrating. However, you may be tempted to remove them by squeezing your skin or using pore strips. It is important to note that these methods can have more negative effects on your skin than positive ones if not done correctly.

With time, you may also result in:

- Peeling
- Dryness
- Irritation
- open pores and infection

Retinol or retinoid-containing topical treatments can aid in maintaining clean, clear pores.

Using an extraction tool is an additional method of getting rid of sebaceous filaments. There is a tiny circle at the end of this little metal instrument.

Having them removed by a dermatologist or esthetician is the safest method. If it's comfortable for you, you can then try this at home:

- Start with a clean face and instrument.
- Always sanitize your instrument with rubbing alcohol before and after use to prevent infections.

+ Gently apply pressure to the bump's circle to check for filament. Be cautious as too much pressure can cause scarring.
+ Treat the area with moisturizer after.

Applying benzoyl peroxide after washing before extraction could also provide further advantages.

3. Scars, blemishes, and hyperpigmentation

It can take a few weeks, six months, or even more in some circumstances for blemishes, scars, and dark areas to heal and vanish. Using cosmetics and sunscreen is part of the immediate therapy for scars and blemishes to prevent future sun damage and hyperpigmentation.

Other ingredients known to help fade scars include:

> **Honey:** According to preliminary research, honey helps heal scars and wounds. When searching for a remedy at home, honey can be of interest. Remember, not just any honey from the grocery store will do, you need medical-grade honey.

- ➤ **Silicone:** Research indicates that applying silicone topically can enhance the thickness, color, and texture of scars. Silicone gel can be used for eight to twenty-four hours per day. Seek for items that list silicon dioxide among their ingredients.

- ➤ **Vitamin C**: When purchasing creams and moisturizers, it is important to pay attention to the ingredients. If vitamin C is dissolved in water and exposed to air or light, it can break down very quickly. That is why a good quality vitamin C product is usually packaged in a brown glass bottle.

Vitamin C works better when combined with other lightening ingredients like soy and licorice

- ➤ **Niacinamide:** Research unequivocally demonstrates that niacinamide is an effective solution for reducing blemishes and dark spots resulting from acne. This is especially true for individuals with lighter skin tones, including those of East Asian origin. It has been scientifically proven that applying niacinamide topically at a concentration of 2-5% can indeed produce positive outcomes.

After cleansing your skin, look for products that include these substances and incorporate them into your routine. Always wear sunscreen after applying it to prevent hyperpigmentation and UV damage.

Chapter 3

How to test your skin type at home

To find out your skin type, you can do a physical test. Sebum production is measured with a home test. Your pores release a waxy, greasy liquid called sebum. Your skin's sebum production level can reveal whether your skin is:

- ❖ dry
- ❖ oily
- ❖ normal
- ❖ combination

The most accurate technique to find out what type of skin you have is to test sebum production on a clean face by following these steps:

1. Wash your face and pat it dry. Wait 30 minutes.

2. Gently press oil blotting paper or tissue on your face. Press the paper on different areas of your

skin, such as your forehead and nose, cheeks, and chin.

3. Apply gentle pressure with oil blotting paper or tissue to various areas of your face, including your forehead, nose, cheeks, and chin.

4. To check the transparency of the paper, hold the sheet up to the light.

Test results	Skin type
Transparency is absent, yet skin tight or covered with flakes	dry
Soaked through	oily
different absorbance values on various facial areas	combination

Not too oily and no flaky skin	normal

In addition to the skin types mentioned above, sensitive skin is another kind that does not meet the sebum criterion. Careful skin is dependent upon:

- how fast your skin reacts to product application
- how easily your skin turns red
- how effectively does your skin shield itself
- Possibility of a skin allergy

Chapter 4

Avoid these do-it-yourself {D I Y} tricks, even if they seem common.

People have reported amazing results when using toothpaste and lemon juice as DIY remedies for common skin issues including dark spots and acne pimples. Emma Stone, an award-winning actress, says baking soda is her secret to good skin.

I just wanted to let you know that some of those skincare hacks you've been trying out may do more harm than good. They might seem like quick fixes, but in reality, they can damage your skin's protective barrier. So, it's important to be careful and gentle with your skin to keep it healthy and glowing.

Avoid these DIY hacks

1. **Sugar:** As an exfoliant, sugar is too harsh for the skin on your face.

2. **Vitamin E:** Topical vitamin E use has the potential to irritate skin and has not been shown to reduce the appearance of scars.

3. **Lemon juice:** Although it contains citric acid, it is far too acidic and can result in the formation of black spots when exposed to the sun. It may also cause skin irritation and drying.

4. **Garlic:** In raw form, garlic can cause skin allergies, eczema, skin inflammation, and watery blisters.

5. Toothpaste is a popular product that is meant to be used for oral hygiene. It is composed of many different ingredients that are designed to clean teeth and freshen breath. Although toothpaste can help kill germs and absorb oil, it is important to note that some of these ingredients can be harsh on your skin. Certain toothpaste ingredients can cause excessive dryness or irritation, particularly if they are applied to sensitive areas. Therefore, it is important to use

toothpaste in moderation and pay attention to any reactions your skin may have to it.

Even while some of these ingredients are inexpensive and all-natural, they aren't made specifically for your skin type.

It's important to understand that some ingredients used in DIY skin care applications can have delayed or long-term effects on your skin, even if you don't notice any immediate side effects. To avoid causing any damage to your skin, it is recommended to use products that are specifically formulated for your face. If you are considering using a DIY skin care product, it's best to talk to your doctor or dermatologist first, to ensure that the ingredients are safe for your skin type and won't cause any harm in the long run.

Putting it all together

You've chosen a few products and performed patch tests on them. After that, you can begin creating a daily routine.

It's important to establish a routine that works for you, but it's also important to recognize that sometimes life gets in the way. You may find it difficult to stick to your routine every day, particularly in situations where you're dealing with illness, fatigue, or traveling without access to your usual products. While it's important to aim for consistency, it's equally important to be flexible and kind to yourself when circumstances prevent you from following your usual routine. Remember, self-care is a journey, and it's okay to deviate from your routine from time to time.

nonetheless, you should at the very least take off your makeup before going to bed and wear sunscreen every day.

Sample routines

one possible routine to try:

1. After waking up: start with a cleanser, then apply spot treatment or serum, followed by moisturizer and sunscreen.

2. The evening routine is the same, except sunscreen is not needed.

Another routine to consider:

1. After waking up, use an antioxidant-rich SPF, a gentle cleanser, and a moisturizer.
2. Before going to bed, use a gentle cleanser, retinol, and moisturizer.

Things to keep in mind

Crafting a personalized skincare routine can be a challenging and time-consuming process. It involves trying out a plethora of different brands and products to discover the ones that are best suited to your unique skin type and concerns. This can involve a bit of trial and error, as not all skin care products will work for everyone. However, with patience and persistence, you can eventually find the right combination of cleansers, exfoliants, toners, serums, moisturizers, and sunscreens that will help you achieve healthy, glowing skin. So, if you're looking to create a perfect skincare routine, be prepared to experiment and be patient in your search for the best products.

Nonetheless, the process can be enjoyable if you don't mind rolling up your sleeves and doing some experimenting.

Additionally, remember that your skin's requirements may change occasionally due to factors beyond your control. Gordon makes this point, which is why you should constantly be aware of your skin.

In case you notice a change in weather or experience dehydration, it's important to provide your skin with extra moisture to keep it healthy and glowing. You can use a moisturizer that suits your skin type to prevent dryness and flakiness. On the other hand, if you happen to experience a breakout or acne, it's advisable to use appropriate acne medication or treatment to help clear your skin. It's always best to consult a dermatologist or healthcare professional to determine the best treatment for your specific skin concern.

Chapter 5

Skin purging

In skin care, purging describes your skin's reaction to new active ingredients.

You might notice:

- dry, peeling skin
- cysts
- whiteheads

If you're having any of the following reactions, you're probably purging:

- appear where outbreaks are usually expected to
- heal more quickly than your average pimples

It's not necessary to discard your new product after purging.

Your skin may be experiencing a reaction to the new ingredients in your skincare products. However, it is important to note that this reaction may be temporary and your skin may simply need a little time to adjust. It is recommended that you wait a few weeks before making any changes to your skincare routine. This will give your skin enough time to adapt and you can observe the results to determine if the new products are working for you or not.

During this period, you must avoid picking at any pimples or blemishes that may appear on your skin, as this can further aggravate the condition. Picking can also lead to scarring and other skin damage, which can be difficult to repair. Instead, try to maintain a regular cleansing routine and use gentle, non-comedogenic products to keep your skin clean and hydrated. This will help to reduce any inflammation or irritation and promote healthy skin.

Some advice to think about while you shop

When it comes to shopping online, it can be quite tempting to search for your favorite products at the lowest possible prices. However, it's important to keep in mind that third-party websites such as Amazon or

Walmart may not always have reliable reviews for the discounted items you come across. While you may be eager to save some money, it's crucial to do your research and ensure that the product you're interested in purchasing has positive feedback and a good reputation among consumers. This will not only ensure your satisfaction with the product but also help you avoid any potential scams or frauds.

For example, you may find reviews where buyers report:

- Damaged packaging
- expired products
- unpleasant or unusual product smell
- products with a different color than usual

To ensure the safety and authenticity of your skincare products, it's important to do your research and find out which sites are authorized to sell a particular brand. Keep in mind that some high-end skincare lines have strict policies that prohibit the sale of their products on certain websites, such as Amazon. Therefore, it's important to double-check the legitimacy of the seller before making a purchase. Opting for unauthorized sellers may put your skin at risk of exposure to counterfeit or expired products, which can cause severe skin reactions and damage. So, take the extra time to verify the authenticity of the seller and their products before making any purchases.

Keep in mind, too, that reviews — while often helpful — can sometimes be deceiving. Brands, for example, frequently post just the greatest product reviews on their website. If you want a more balanced viewpoint, consider searching Google for additional product reviews.

When you're reading product reviews online, it's important to dig deeper and look into the source of the reviews. One factor to consider is whether the reviews are coming from social media influencers. While these influencers can provide valuable insights into a product, it's important to keep in mind that they may have a vested interest in promoting a particular brand or product. This doesn't necessarily mean that their review is false or misleading, but it's something to keep in mind when evaluating the credibility of the review. It's always a good idea to read multiple reviews from different sources to get a well-rounded understanding of a product before making a purchase decision.

If you see a sponsored review, examine other reviews before making a decision.

It's always a good idea to consider your budget before embarking on a shopping spree. It's easy to get carried away and overspend, but being mindful of your financial limitations can help you make wiser purchasing decisions. Keep in mind that just because something is expensive doesn't necessarily mean it's of higher quality or better suited to your needs. Take your time to compare prices and read reviews before making your final purchase, and don't hesitate to opt for more affordable options that are still of good quality and fit your requirements.

Chapter 6

When to Consult a Dermatologist

Are you feeling overwhelmed by the vast selection of skincare products available? Are you unsure of your skin's unique needs?

A dermatologist can provide more individualized guidance on how to formulate the best skincare routine.

the value of consulting a dermatologist if you have several skin issues. They can assist you in creating a focused treatment plan.

If you are looking to improve the health and appearance of your skin, seeking support from a dermatologist can be extremely beneficial. However, it is important to note that accessing professional help may not always be possible due to various reasons such as financial constraints, lack of availability, or time constraints. In such cases, a good starting point would be to opt for a limited assortment of gentle or mild skin care products.

These products are usually formulated to be less irritating and are therefore less likely to cause adverse reactions.

It is important to note that everyone's skin is different and may react differently to different products. Therefore, it is advisable to start with a small range of products and gradually add to them over time as needed. This will allow you to monitor how your skin reacts to specific products and make adjustments accordingly. Remember, consistency is key when it comes to skincare, so sticking to a routine that works for you is essential in achieving optimal results.

Conclusion

Developing a customized skincare routine can go a long way in keeping your skin looking radiant and healthy. To begin with, it's important to identify your skin type and the specific goals you wish to achieve through your skin care regimen. For instance, if you're looking to address issues such as dryness, acne, or fine lines, you may need to incorporate specific products and ingredients into your routine. Consulting with a dermatologist or a skincare expert can also help determine the optimal routine for your skin type and concerns. With the right combination of products, tailored to your specific needs, you can achieve smoother, clearer, and more youthful-looking skin.

When it comes to taking care of your skin, it's important to remember that a little patience can go a long way. This is particularly true when trying new skincare ingredients or waiting for results. It's best to introduce new products slowly, starting with a patch test, and gradually increasing the frequency and amount of product used. This can help prevent any adverse reactions or irritations.

Additionally, if you have any persistent skin concerns, it's always a good idea to reach out to a dermatologist for professional advice. They can help diagnose any underlying skin conditions and recommend appropriate treatments or skincare routines. Remember, taking care of your skin is a long-term commitment, and it's important to approach it with patience, diligence, and expert guidance.